The Ultimate Yoga Guide for senior women

A Genl'le Approach I'o Yoga for Senior Women: Mind, Body, and Spiril'"

BY

FELIX RICH

TABLE OF CONTENT

Introduction

Chapter One

Why yoga is Beneficial for senior women

Safety Considerations for senior women

Chapter Two

Getting started with yoga

Chapter Three

Basic yoga poses for senior women

Chapter Four

Yoga sequences for senior women

Among the many yoga benefits for women
Additional Information

Introduction

Yoga can help senior women enhance their entire health and well-being safely and effectively. Our bodies grow less flexible as we age, our joints stiffen, and our balance may suffer. Yoga can help with these problems by increasing flexibility, balance, and mobility.

It is important to note, however, that not all yoga poses are appropriate for older ladies. It's critical to locate a yoga instructor who understands the requirements and limits of senior ladies. This will allow them to reap the advantages of yoga while avoiding harm.

It is critical to select a yoga guide for senior ladies that prioritizes safety and accessibility.

Gentle, low-impact positions that are easy on the joints, such as seated or reclining poses, should be included in the guide. The guide should also provide adjustments for persons with limited mobility or physical restrictions.

Yoga has various advantages for senior women. Yoga can help you improve your flexibility, and strength, reduce tension and anxiety, and sleep better. Yoga has also been demonstrated to help reduce chronic pain symptoms and enhance overall mood and well-being.

Senior women should contact their healthcare physician before beginning any new fitness routine. Once they've received the all-clear, they may begin their yoga practice with confidence, knowing that they're doing something good for their health and well-being.

Finally, yoga is a risk-free and effective technique for older women to improve their entire health and well-being. Finding a yoga guide who is sensitive to the requirements and limits of senior women can help them reap the benefits of yoga while avoiding injury. Senior women can improve their flexibility, strength, stress, anxiety levels, and sleep quality with frequent practice.

Chapter one

Why Yoga is Beneficial for senior women

Yoga is a fantastic kind of exercise for senior ladies since it provides several physical, mental, and emotional benefits. Here are some of the ways that senior ladies can benefit from yoga practice:

A. **Improves flexibility and mobility:** As we get older, our muscles and joints stiffen and become less flexible. Regular yoga practice can help improve flexibility and range of motion, making everyday actions like bending, reaching, and twisting easier.

B. **Strengthens and improves balance:** Many yoga poses require you to hold yourself in various positions, which can help you build strength and improve your balance. This is especially critical for senior women, who are more prone to falls and fractures.

C. **Yoga has been demonstrated to lower stress and anxiety:** which can be especially good for senior women who may be suffering from a variety of physical and emotional issues.

D. **Yoga has been shown to promote heart health:** by lowering blood pressure and lowering the risk of heart disease. This is especially critical for elderly women, who are predisposed to heart disease as they age.

E. **Improves mental clarity and attention:** Yoga can assist enhance mental clarity and focus, which can be good for senior women experiencing cognitive loss.

F. **Improves sleep:** Yoga can assist improve sleep by lowering stress and encouraging relaxation. This is especially crucial for senior women who may have difficulty sleeping owing to a variety of medical issues or drugs.

In summary, yoga can be an excellent kind of exercise for senior women, providing numerous physical, mental, and emotional benefits. It is critical to work with a professional yoga instructor who can provide modifications and adaptations for any physical limits or health concerns.

Safety Considerations for senior women

Yoga can be a safe and effective activity for older women, but certain precautions must be taken to avoid injury and ensure a happy experience. Here are some safety precautions for senior ladies who practice yoga:

01. **Consult with a healthcare provider:** As with any new workout regimen, it's vital to check with your doctor to confirm that yoga is safe for you.

02. **Practice under the supervision of a competent instructor:** A qualified instructor may assist you in modifying poses to meet your specific requirements and abilities, as well as provide advice on proper alignment and breathing methods.

03. **Use props:** Props like blocks, blankets, and straps can assist you adjust poses and provide extra support.

04. **Avoid overstretching:** Because our muscles become less flexible as we age, it's critical to avoid overstretching and pushing yourself beyond your limits. Concentrate on progressively developing your flexibility over time.

05. **Exercise with awareness:** Consider your body and how it feels in each stance. Back off or alter the stance as needed if you experience pain or discomfort.

06. **Consider chair yoga:** For senior ladies who have trouble getting up and down from the floor, chair yoga can be a terrific option. It enables you to perform yoga while seated or supported by a chair.

07. **Select a secure environment:** Check that the yoga studio or class is well-lit, clear of obstructions, and has a non-slip surface.

Senior women can get the numerous physical, mental, and emotional advantages of yoga by following these safety precautions.

Chapter Two

Getting started with yoga

Yoga is an excellent approach to increasing flexibility, balance, and general physical and mental health. Here are some basic steps to getting started with yoga:

1. **Set your intention:** Before you begin practicing yoga, you should think about what you want to achieve. This might range from increasing flexibility to lowering tension and anxiety.

2. **Choose a style:** There are numerous yoga styles, each with its distinct focus and advantages. Hatha, Vinyasa, Bikram, and

Yin are popular styles. Spend some time researching different styles to discover one that speaks to you.

3. **Find a teacher or class:** As a beginner, it is beneficial to have an experienced teacher assist you through your yoga practice. Look for a yoga studio or gym in your area, or find an online teacher or class to follow along with.

4. **Get the proper equipment:** While no particular equipment is required to perform yoga, knowing the fundamentals is beneficial. A comfortable mat is required, and depending on the kind of yoga you choose, you may want to invest in blocks, straps, and other props to help support your practice.

5. **Begin with basic poses:** As a beginner, it is critical, to begin with, basic yoga poses to develop a firm foundation. Some excellent poses

6. **Regular practice:** Yoga, like any other kind of exercise, requires constancy. To reap the best benefits, practice at least a couple of times every week.

Remember that yoga is a personal practice, so don't worry about being perfect or comparing yourself to others. Simply listen to your body and do what feels comfortable to you.

Chapter Three

Basic yoga poses for senior women

Yoga can be an excellent type of exercise for senior ladies, improving flexibility, balance, and overall health. However, it is critical to select positions that are both safe and appropriate for your body. Here are some mild and appropriate yoga positions for senior women:

- **Tadasana (Mountain Pose):**

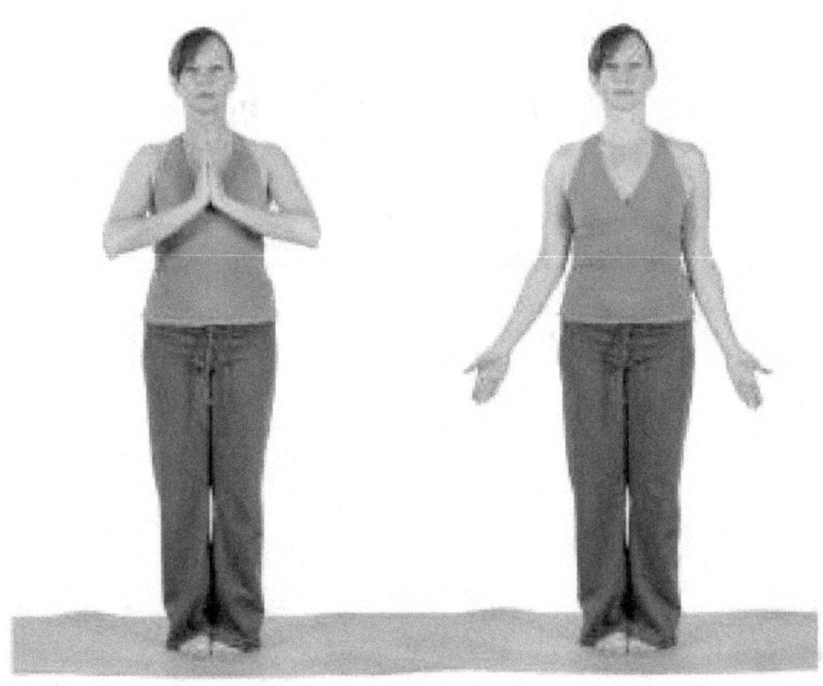

This is a basic standing pose that can help improve posture and balance. Stand with your feet hip-width apart, your toes pointed forward, and your arms at your sides relaxed. Concentrate on anchoring your feet and stretching your spine.

- **Cat/Cow Pose (Marjaryasana/Bitilasana):**

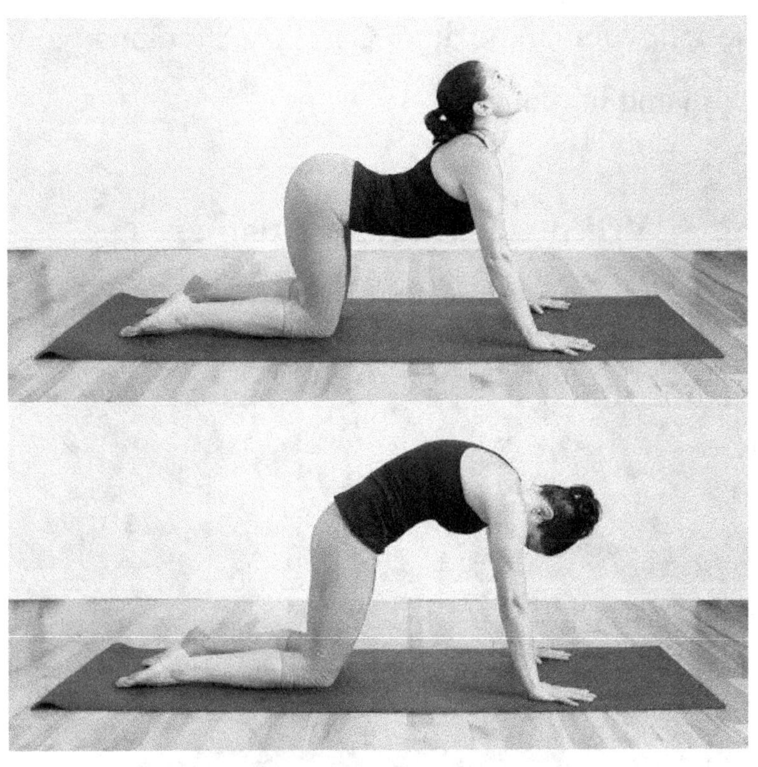

This smooth transition between two poses can aid in spinal mobilization and flexibility. Begin on your hands and knees, wrists directly under your shoulders, and knees directly under your hips. Inhale and arch your spine into Cow Pose, elevating your head and tailbone. Exhale and round your spine into Cat Pose, tucking your chin and tailbone.

- **Vrikshasana (Tree position):**

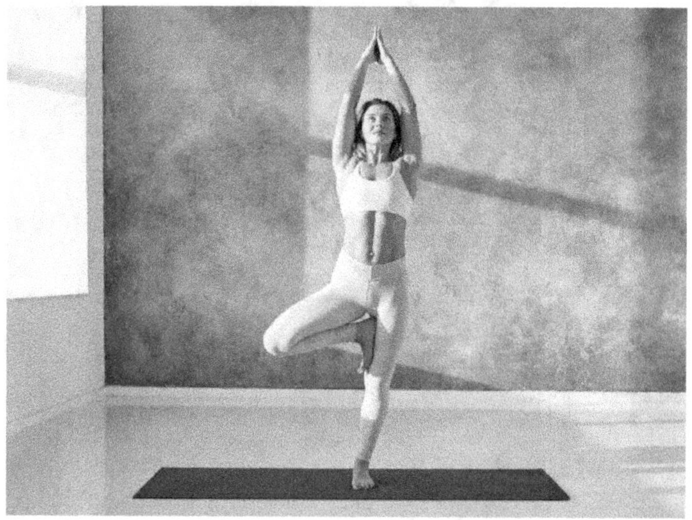

This position can aid with balance and stability. Start in Mountain Pose and then move your weight to your left foot. Avoid placing your right foot directly on the knee by placing it on your left ankle, calf, or thigh. Bring your hands to the middle of your chest or stretch your arms upwards.

- **Warrior II (Virabhadrasana II):**

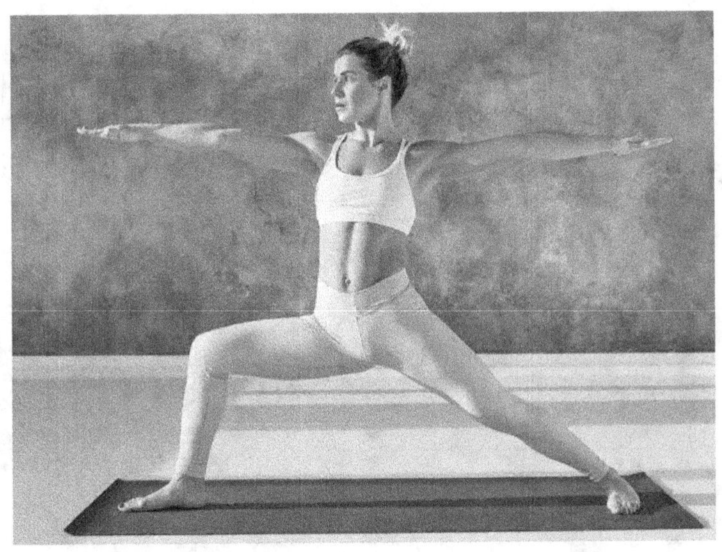

This pose can assist in increasing leg and hip strength and stability. Begin in Mountain Pose, then take a 3-4 foot step back with your left foot. Make a 90-degree angle with your left foot and a 90-degree angle with your right knee. Extend your arms to the sides and look down at your right fingertips.

Seated Forward Fold (Paschimottanasana):

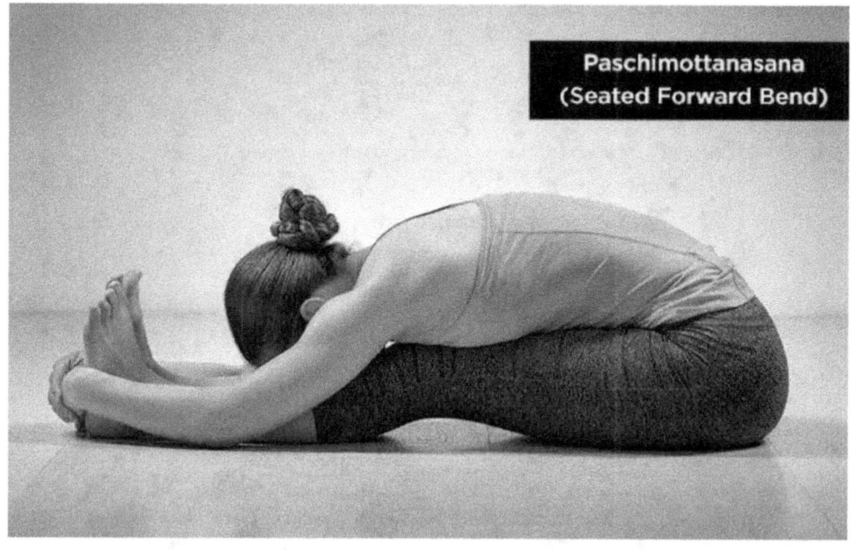

This pose can aid in the increased hamstring and lower back flexibility. Sit on the floor, legs straight out in front of you. Inhale deeply and extend your arms upwards, stretching your spine. Exhale and swing your hips forward, bringing your hands towards your feet or ankles.

Always listen to your body and do only what is comfortable and safe for you. Before beginning a yoga practice, contact your doctor or a trained yoga teacher if you have any concerns or health conditions.

Chapter Four

Yoga sequences for senior women

Yoga is a great way for senior women to improve their flexibility, balance, and overall health. Here are some yoga exercises that are suitable for senior women:

→ **Moderate Warm-up Sequence**

This sequence is appropriate for seniors who are new to yoga or who want a gentle warm-up before engaging in a more intense practice.

Begin with a few rounds of simple neck stretches that involve rotating your head in circles and from side to side.

To accomplish shoulder rolls, move your shoulders forward and backward.

Then, cross your legs and gently twist to the right and left.

Finally, reach your hands to your feet and hold the stretch for a few breaths.

→ Routine for Chair Yoga:

If you have limited movement or balance issues, chair yoga could be a great option.

Sit in a chair with your feet flat on the ground and your hands on your thighs. Take a few deep breaths.

Raise your arms and stretch them towards the ceiling. Bend forward at the waist and reach your hands to the ground.

Place your hands on your knees and gradually twist your body while looking over your shoulder.

Finish with some seated stretches, such as stretching your arms behind your back and clasping your hands.

→ **Standing balance sequence:**

This sequence helps build balance and stability.

Start in a mountain stance, with your feet hip-width apart and your arms by your sides.

Lift your right leg and place your foot on your left thigh to enter the tree pose. Take a few deep breaths before switching sides.

Then, in Warriorrior 3 position, raise your arms ahead and extend your left leg behind you. Take a few deep breaths before switching sides.

Finally, come into a forward fold while standing, stretching your hands towards the ground and holding for a few breaths.

Always listen to your body and do what feels right. If you have any medical concerns or limitations, talk to your doctor before starting a new workout routine.

Chapter Five

Breathing Techniques for senior women

Pranayama, or breathing methods, is an essential aspect of yoga practice. They can assist senior women in reducing stress, increasing lung capacity, and improving their general sense of well-being. Here are some breathing strategies for senior women who practice yoga:

1) Deep breathing:

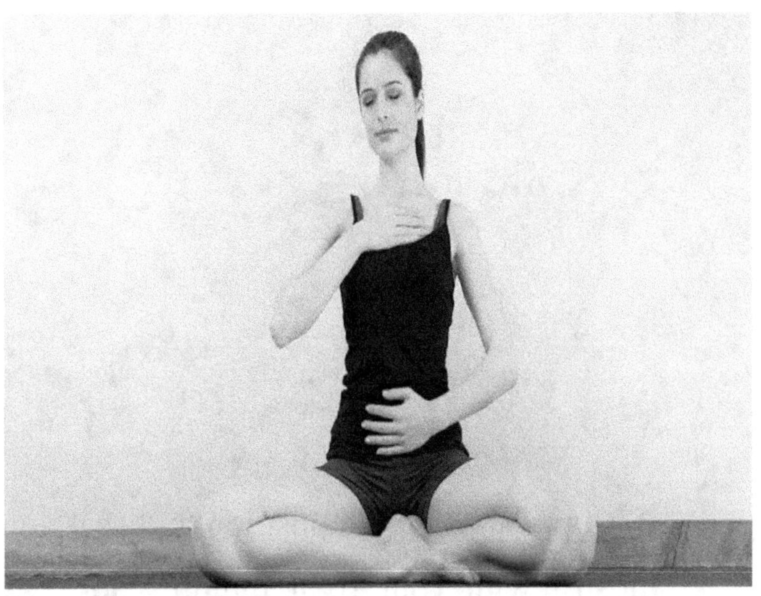

Sit in a comfortable position and place your hands on your abdomen to practice abdominal breathing. Deeply inhale through your nose, feeling your stomach rise as you fill your lungs with air. Exhale through your nose, feeling your abdomen drop as you let the breath out of your lungs. Continue for a few minutes.

2) Alternate Nostril Breathing:

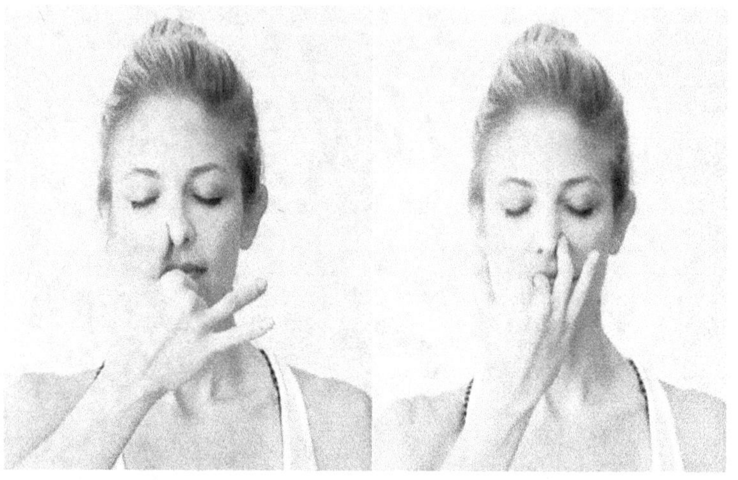

Sit in a comfortable position and seal your right nostril with your right thumb. Close your left nostril with your right index finger after inhaling through it. Hold your breath for a few seconds, then exhale through your right nostril. Repeat for a few minutes before switching to your left nostril.

3) Three-part breathing:

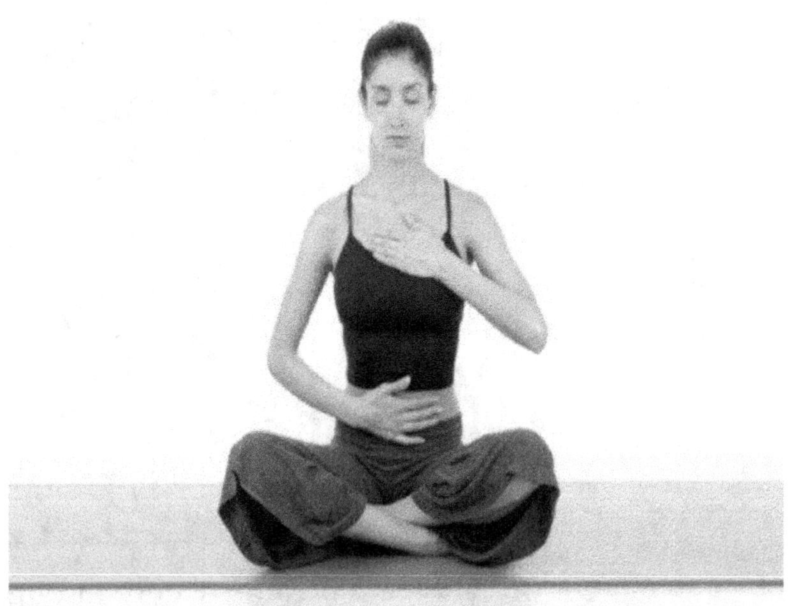

Sit in a comfortable position and rest your hands on your abdomen, ribcage, and chest. Inhale deeply and fill your lower abdomen, then your ribs, and lastly your chest with air. Exhale in the opposite sequence, first from your chest, then from your ribcage, and finally from your abdomen. Repeat a few times.

4) Ujjayi Breath:

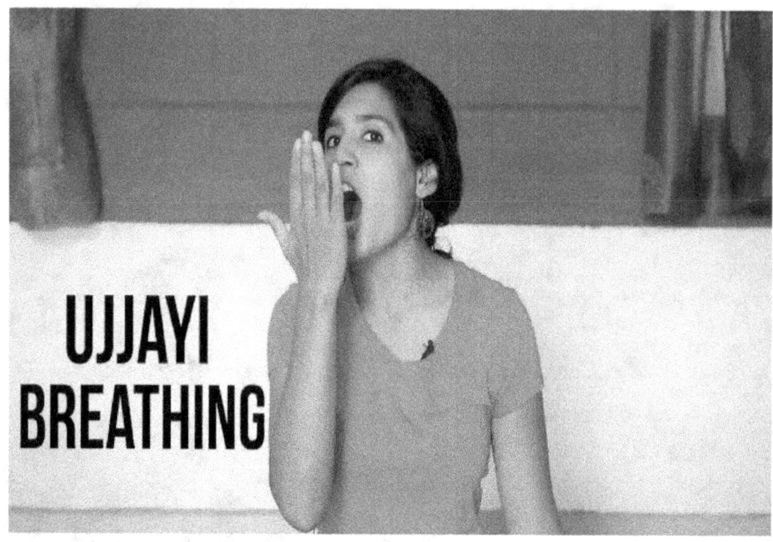

Sit comfortably and breathe deeply through your nose. Exhale through your mouth, tightening your neck and generating a quiet "ha" sound. Continue for a few minutes.

5) Lions breath:

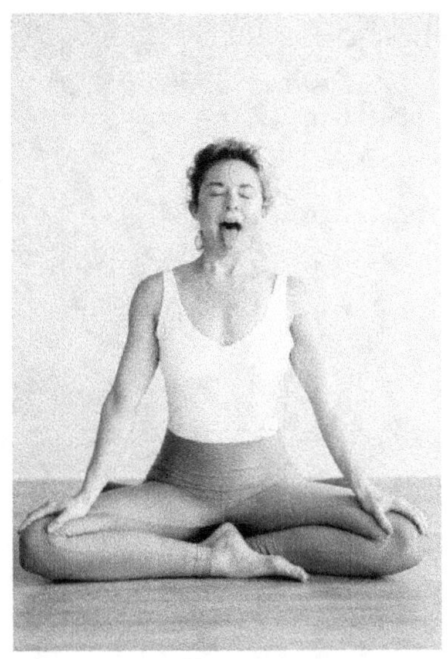

Sit in a comfortable position and breathe deeply through your nose. Exhale by opening your mouth wide and sticking out your tongue to make a "roar" sound. Continue for a few minutes.

It's critical to remember to listen to your body and not overwork yourself. Stop immediately and seek the advice of a trained yoga teacher if you experience any discomfort or pain while performing any of these methods.

Chapter Six

Meditation and relaxation techniques for senior women

Meditation and relaxation practices can help older women who practice yoga reduce stress, develop mindfulness, and promote general well-being. Here are a few techniques that might be useful:

Encourage seniors to take long, slow, deep breaths through their noses, filling their abdomen and lungs with air before gently exhaling through their mouths. This can assist to alleviate tension and anxiety while also increasing attention and concentration.

Yoga Nidra, often known as "yogic sleep," is a deep relaxation method that can help seniors relieve stress and sleep better. It entails lying down in a comfortable position and listening to a guided meditation that focuses on various regions of the body, breathing, and vision.

Body Scan: This relaxation technique is slowly scanning the body from head to toe, focusing on each portion of the body and intentionally relaxing any stiff or tight places. This can assist seniors in releasing physical and mental strain as well as increasing body awareness.

Guided imagery is the visualization of calming scenes, such as a peaceful beach or a tranquil forest. This can assist elders in reducing stress, increasing relaxation, and encouraging positive thinking.

Mindfulness Meditation entails paying attention to the present moment and monitoring thoughts and feelings without judgment. It can assist elders in increasing alertness, decreasing tension, and promoting mental clarity.

Overall, seniors should be encouraged to find approaches that work for them and to approach meditation and relaxation with an open mind and curiosity.

Chapter Seven

Common medical issues and how yoga could potentially help

There are numerous common health difficulties that people may face, and yoga can be a helpful practice in managing or alleviating symptoms related to these concerns. Here are a couple of such examples:

1. **Anxiety:** Yoga can help relieve stress and anxiety by boosting relaxation and decreasing the production of stress hormones like cortisol. Mindfulness and breath control practices can assist to calm the mind and increase mental clarity.

2. **Back Pain:** By strengthening the muscles that support the spine and improving posture, yoga can help relieve back pain. Poses including a downward-facing dog, cat-cow, and child's pose can help stretch and release back stress.

3. **Insomnia:** Yoga can help with insomnia by lowering stress and encouraging relaxation. Forward bends and inversions can also assist to relax the mind and prepare the body for sleep.

4. **Arthritis:** Yoga can help with cardiovascular health by lowering blood pressure, boosting circulation, and enhancing heart function. Vinyasa or

power yoga, for example, can also give a cardiovascular workout.

5. **Depression:** Yoga can help manage depression symptoms by lowering stress and encouraging relaxation. It can also help with mood enhancement by raising the synthesis of feel-good chemicals like serotonin and dopamine.

In summary, yoga has several benefits for both physical and mental health. Always consult with a healthcare provider before beginning a new training regimen, especially if you have any pre-existing health concerns.

Chapter eight

Frequently Asked Questions about Senior Women's Yoga

Here are some frequently asked questions about senior women's yoga:

Is yoga suitable for elderly women?

Yes, yoga can be safe and good for elderly women, but before beginning any new exercise program, consult with your doctor. It is also critical to select a yoga instructor who has been trained to deal with elders and can adjust poses to meet any physical restrictions.

What are the advantages of yoga for older women?

Yoga can assist senior women in maintaining flexibility, improving balance, decreasing tension, and promoting relaxation. Chronic illnesses such as arthritis, osteoporosis, and back pain can also benefit from it.

What styles of yoga are most suitable for senior women?

For older women, gentle yoga, chair yoga, and restorative yoga are all viable possibilities. These yoga methods are slower-paced and emphasize relaxation and mild stretching.

What should senior ladies wear to yoga?

Comfortable, loose-fitting clothing with a full range of motion is ideal. Avoid wearing clothing that is overly tight or constricting. It is also critical to wear comfy shoes or none at all.

Do I need any special equipment for yoga?

No, no particular equipment is required to perform yoga. A yoga mat is useful but not required. Props such as yoga blocks, belts, and blankets can be used to modify postures if you have any physical constraints.

How frequently should older ladies practice yoga?

The frequency with which yoga is practiced is determined by the individual's health and fitness levels. Yoga should be practiced at least two to three times a week as a general guideline.

Can yoga relieve menopausal symptoms?

Yes, yoga can help with menopausal symptoms such as hot flashes, sleeplessness, and mood swings. Certain yoga positions and breathing methods can aid in the regulation of menopausal hormonal changes.

Always with your doctor before beginning any new exercise regimen, especially if you have any pre-existing medical ailments or concerns.

CHAPTER NINE

Conclusion and more resources

Conclusion

Yoga is a holistic activity with several benefits for women. It helps women build physical strength and flexibility while also lowering tension and anxiety, enhancing mental clarity and focus, and promoting overall well-being. Yoga can also assist women in connecting with their bodies and emotions, thereby bringing balance and harmony into their life.

Among the many special yoga benefits for women are:

1) Eliminating menstrual cramps and PMS symptoms

2) Preparing for childbirth and relieving pregnancy-related pain

3) promoting postpartum healing and recovery

4) Breast health and lymphatic flow are aided.

5) Bone density enhancement and osteoporosis prevention

6) Menopausal symptoms relief

7) Self-acceptance and body positivity cultivation

Women can begin practicing yoga by visiting a class at a local studio, using an online video or app, or practicing at home with this book or DVD. It is critical to listen to your body and select a practice that feels safe and comfortable to you.

Additional information:

Yoga Journal - This website offers a wealth of information on yoga for women, including pose guides, sequences, and articles on specific topics like pregnancy yoga and menopause.

Yoga International - This site offers online classes, articles, and resources for yoga practitioners of all levels, including women's health topics.

Yoga Alliance - This organization offers a directory of certified yoga teachers and studios, as well as information on yoga teacher training programs.

The Woman's Book of Yoga and Health by Linda Sparrowe - This book offers a comprehensive guide to yoga for women's health, including specific sequences for different stages of life.

Yoga for Women by Shakta Kaur Khalsa - This book offers Kundalini yoga practices and meditations specifically designed for women.

www.ingramcontent.com/pod-product-compliance
Lightning Source LLC
Chambersburg PA
CBHW051923250726
48659CB00002B/799